DUMBBELL EXERCISES FOR WOMEN

Shape Your Body, Strengthen Your Mind; A Guide to Effective Dumbbell Training, Targeted Workouts and Sculpting Techniques for Women

Rae A. Lake

TABLE OF CONTENTS

INTRODUCTION 4

CHAPTER I: DUMBBELL TRAINING FOR WOMEN.................7

Benefits of Dumbbell Training for Women 7

Importance of Mind-Body Connection......................9

CHAPTER II: UNDERSTANDING DUMBBELL EXERCISES.....11

Types of Dumbbells 11

How to Choose the Right Dumbbells........................13

Safety Tips for Dumbbell Training 15

Warm-Up and Cool-Down Techniques......................16

Importance of Proper Form....................................18

CHAPTER III: TOTAL BODY WORKOUTS 20

Upper Body Workouts..20

Dumbbell Shoulder Press 20

Dumbbell Flys 21

Dumbbell Lat Pulldowns.....................................21

Dumbbell Bent Over Rows 22

Dumbbell Chest Press..23

Dumbbell Upright Rows 24

Dumbbell Rear Delt Flys 25

Dumbbell Lateral Raises 26

Dumbbell Front Delt Raises 26

Dumbbell Overhead Tricep Extensions 27

Lower Body Workouts 28

Dumbbell Squats 28

Dumbbell Lunges 29

Dumbbell Sumo Squats 30

Dumbbell Hamstring Curls...31

Dumbbell Step-Ups..31

Dumbbell Calf Raises 32

Dumbbell Side Lunges 33

Dumbbell Box Jumps 34

Dumbbell Box Squats...34

Dumbbell Plié Squats 35

Dumbbell Fire Hydrants..36

Core Workouts 37

Dumbbell Side Plank..38

Dumbbell Sit-Ups..38

Dumbbell Leg Raises..39

Dumbbell Plank Holds 40

Dumbbell Scissor Kicks 41

Dumbbell Woodchoppers 42

Dumbbell Leg Lifts 43

Dumbbell Bicycles 44

Dumbbell Reverse Sit-Ups 45

Dumbbell Toe Touches 46

Dumbbell Spiderman Plank 48

Full-Body Workouts 49

Dumbbell Squat and Press..49

Dumbbell Lunges with Bicep Curls 50

Dumbbell Plank to Push-Up......................................50

Dumbbell Russian Twists 51

Dumbbell Clean and Jerk..53

Dumbbell Bulgarian Split Squats 54

Dumbbell Reverse Flys 55

Dumbbell Mountain Climbers 56

Dumbbell Thruster 57

Dumbbell Squat Jumps 58

CHAPTER IV: TARGETED WORKOUTS 60

Arms and Shoulders 60

Dumbbell Bicep Curls 60

Dumbbell Tricep Extensions 61

Dumbbell Hammer Curls 62

Dumbbell Shrugs 63

Dumbbell Pullovers 63

Dumbbell Concentration Curls 64

Dumbbell Close Grip Bench Press 65

Dumbbell Alternating Curls 66

Dumbbell Skull Crushers...67

Chest and Back 68

Dumbbell Bench Press...69

Dumbbell Pullover 69

Dumbbell Row 70

Dumbbell Pull-Up 71

Dumbbell Chest Fly..72

Dumbbell Pulling Kneeling Rows 73

Dumbbell Seated Rows..74

Dumbbell Deadlifts..74

Dumbbell Power Cleans 75

Dumbbell Hang Cleans 76

Legs and Glutes 78

Dumbbell Donkey Kicks 78

Dumbbell Figure Four Stretch 78

Dumbbell Skater Hops...79

Dumbbell Bulgarian Split Squats 80

Dumbbell Glute Bridges...81

Abs and Core 82

Plank Dumbbell Rows..82

Dumbbell Leg Raises..83

Dumbbell Side Bends...84

Dumbbell Reverse Crunches......................................85

Dumbbell Bicycle Crunches 86

Dumbbell Ab Rollouts...87

CHAPTER V: SCULPTING TECHNIQUES 1..89

High-Intensity Interval Training (HIIT) 89

Progressive Overload 90

Supersets and Dropsets...92

Plyometrics...94

CHAPTER VI: MINDFUL TRAINING 96

Mindful Breathing Techniques 96

Visualization and Affirmations for Improved Performance..........101

Final Thoughts 104

Continuing Your Dumbbell Journey...105

INTRODUCTION

Dumbbell exercises have been a staple of strength training for decades, providing a simple and effective way to increase strength, build muscle, and improve overall fitness. Women, in particular, can benefit greatly from incorporating dumbbell exercises into their workout routine. However, many women are intimidated by the idea of lifting weights, or simply don't know where to start. This book was written with the goal of making dumbbell exercises accessible and approachable for women of all fitness levels.

Dumbbell exercises are a versatile and effective way to improve your physical fitness and strength. Whether you are a beginner or an experienced fitness enthusiast, dumbbells can be an essential tool in achieving your fitness goals. Women, in particular, can benefit greatly from incorporating dumbbell training into their fitness routine. Dumbbells offer a wide range of exercises that target specific muscle groups and can help improve strength, endurance, metabolism, balance, and coordination, as well as reduce stress and improve mood.

The benefits of dumbbell training for women are numerous, but the key is to understand how to use dumbbells effectively and safely. This book, *"Dumbbell Exercises for Women"* is designed to help women of all ages and fitness levels unlock the power of dumbbell training and improve their physical fitness and well-being.

Here, you will learn about the benefits of dumbbell training, the types of dumbbells and essential equipment, how to choose the right dumbbells, and safety tips for dumbbell training. We will cover warm-up and cool-down techniques, as well as proper form, and stretching techniques to help you get started on the right foot.

The book includes a variety of total body workouts, targeted workouts, and sculpting techniques to help you achieve your fitness goals. Whether you want to work on your arms and shoulders, chest and back, legs and glutes, or abs and core, this book has a workout for you. We will also discuss high-intensity interval training (HIIT), progressive overload, supersets, dropsets, and plyometrics, among other advanced techniques, to help you continue to challenge yourself as you progress in your fitness journey.

We encourage you to take the time to read this book carefully, to ask questions, and to practice the exercises and techniques described. With time and dedication, you will be able to unlock the power of dumbbell training and achieve the results you desire.

CHAPTER I: DUMBBELL TRAINING FOR WOMEN

Benefits of Dumbbell Training for Women

One of the primary benefits of dumbbell training for women is improved strength and endurance. Dumbbells allow you to target specific muscle groups and provide resistance that helps build strength and tone your muscles. This increased strength can help you perform daily tasks with ease and reduce your risk of injury. In addition, incorporating dumbbells into your workout routine can also improve your endurance, allowing you to perform longer and more intense exercises without fatigue.

Another benefit of dumbbell training for women is increased metabolism. Dumbbells can help you burn more calories and increase your metabolism, which can aid in weight loss. The resistance provided by the dumbbells can also help you build lean muscle mass, which burns more calories than fat, even when you are at rest. This can help you maintain your weight loss and improve your overall health.

Better balance and coordination are also important benefits of dumbbell training for women. The use of dumbbells can help you improve your balance and coordination by targeting specific muscle groups and challenging your stability. This can reduce your risk of falls and improve your overall fitness level. In addition, incorporating balance exercises into your dumbbell training can help you develop better posture and body control, which can help you avoid pain and discomfort in your daily life.

Reduced stress and improved mood are two additional benefits of dumbbell training for women. Exercise has been shown to release endorphins, which are natural mood-boosting chemicals in the body. In addition, the physical exertion and focus required during a dumbbell workout can help you relieve stress and improve your overall mood. Exercise has also been shown to improve sleep, which can help you feel refreshed and energized during the day.

Finally, increased bone density is a crucial benefit of dumbbell training for women. As women age, their bone density decreases, increasing their risk of osteoporosis. Dumbbell training can help build bone density and reduce the risk of osteoporosis. This can improve your overall health and reduce the risk of fractures and falls as you age.

Importance of Mind-Body Connection

The importance of mind-body connection is often overlooked when it comes to fitness and exercise. However, it is a critical aspect of reaching one's fitness goals and ensuring a healthy and balanced lifestyle. Mind-body connection refers to the integration of physical and mental awareness during exercise, which can help improve both the physical and mental outcomes of exercise.

One of the key benefits of mind-body connection is improved focus and concentration. By focusing on the movements and sensations in your body, you are able to tune out distractions and stay present in the moment. This improved focus can help you perform exercises more effectively, reducing the risk of injury and allowing you to push your limits further.

In addition, mind-body connection can help reduce stress and anxiety. Exercise is already well known for its stress-relieving properties, but incorporating mindfulness into your workout can enhance these benefits. When you are focused on the physical sensations in your body, you are less likely to be caught up in worries and thoughts, which can help to reduce stress and anxiety levels.

Another benefit of mind-body connection is increased self-awareness. By paying attention to the way your body feels during exercise, you can become more aware of any imbalances or areas of tightness, which can help you to target those areas in your workouts. This increased self-awareness can also help you to identify any physical limitations that may be holding you back and find ways to overcome them.

Finally, mind-body connection can help to improve your overall enjoyment of exercise. When you are fully present and focused on the sensations in your body, you are more likely to experience a sense of flow and enjoyment during your workout. This can help to create a positive association with exercise, making it easier to stick to your workout routine in the long-term.

CHAPTER II: UNDERSTANDING DUMBBELL EXERCISES

Types of Dumbbells

Dumbbells are a versatile and convenient piece of equipment that can be used for a variety of strength training exercises. There are several different types of dumbbells, each with its own unique features and benefits.

Fixed Dumbbells: These are the traditional type of dumbbells, where the weight plates are permanently attached to the bar. They come in a variety of weight sizes, making them a great choice for individuals who want to gradually increase the weight they are lifting.

Adjustable Dumbbells: As the name suggests, adjustable dumbbells can be adjusted to different weight sizes, making them a versatile and convenient choice for those who want to save space and time. They usually consist of a bar and a set of weight plates that can be added or removed as needed.

Kettlebells: Kettlebells are similar to traditional dumbbells, but they have a handle that is attached to a weight. They are typically used for explosive movements such as swings and snatches, making them a great choice for those looking to increase their power and explosiveness.

Selectorized Dumbbells: Selectorized dumbbells are a type of adjustable dumbbell that uses a selector pin to change the weight. They are easy to use and can be adjusted quickly, making them a great choice for those who want to switch between exercises quickly.

Each type of dumbbell has its own unique features and benefits, and the best type for you will depend on your specific fitness goals and the type of exercises you want to do. In this book, we will explore the different types of dumbbells in more detail and help you choose the right type for your needs.

In addition to Dumbbells, there are several other essential pieces of equipment that can help you get the most out of your strength training routine. Some of these include:

Resistance Bands: Resistance bands are a versatile and portable piece of equipment that can be used for a variety of exercises, including upper body, lower body, and core workouts. They come in a variety of resistance levels, making them a great choice for individuals of all fitness levels.

Yoga Mat: A yoga mat is an essential piece of equipment for many strength training exercises, as it provides a comfortable and supportive surface to perform exercises on. It also helps to protect your joints and reduce the risk of injury.

Foam Roller: A foam roller is a great tool for stretching and self-massage, and can help to improve flexibility and relieve muscle tightness and pain.

Stability Ball: A stability ball is a versatile piece of equipment that can be used for a variety of exercises, including upper body, lower body, and core workouts. It can also be used for balance and stability exercises, making it a great choice for individuals looking to improve their balance and coordination.

How to Choose the Right Dumbbells

Choosing the right dumbbells for your strength training routine is important for ensuring that you get the most out of your workouts and avoid injury. Here are some factors to consider when choosing your dumbbells:

Weight: The weight of your dumbbells will depend on your current fitness level, strength, and the type of exercises you will be performing. It's best to start with lighter weights and gradually increase the weight as you progress in your strength training journey.

Adjustability: Adjustable dumbbells are a great option for those who want to switch between different weights during a single workout. They are also more space-efficient and cost-effective compared to purchasing multiple sets of fixed weight dumbbells.

Material: Dumbbells come in a variety of materials, including rubber, neoprene, and cast iron. Each material has its own benefits, so it's important to consider the type of exercises you will be performing, as well as the environment in which you will be using the dumbbells.

Comfort: The comfort and grip of your dumbbells is important, especially if you will be using them for extended periods of time. Look for dumbbells with comfortable grips and ergonomic design to avoid discomfort and injury.

By considering these factors, you can choose the right dumbbells for your strength training routine and achieve your fitness goals.

Safety Tips for Dumbbell Training

Safety is always a top priority when it comes to strength training, especially when using dumbbells. Here are some important safety tips to keep in mind:

Warm up: Before starting your strength training routine, it's important to warm up to prepare your muscles and joints for the workout ahead. This can include light cardio exercises, stretching, or foam rolling.

Proper form: Maintaining proper form during exercises is essential to avoiding injury. Make sure to align your body and engage the right muscles while performing exercises with dumbbells.

Progress gradually: Don't try to lift too much weight too soon. Gradually increase the weight as you progress in your strength training journey, and avoid pushing yourself too hard too soon.

Use a spotter: When performing exercises with heavy weights, it's a good idea to have a spotter assist you. This can help to avoid injury and ensure that you are lifting with proper form.

Warm down: After your strength training routine, it's important to cool down and stretch your muscles to prevent stiffness and injury.

By following these safety tips, you can minimize the risk of injury and get the most out of your dumbbell training routine.

Warm-Up and Cool-Down Techniques

Warm-up and cool-down techniques are essential components of any strength training routine, including those that involve dumbbells. Here are some tips for effective warm-up and cool-down techniques:

Warm-Up:

Light cardio: Start your workout with 5-10 minutes of light cardio exercises, such as jogging or jumping jacks, to increase your heart rate and get your blood flowing.

Dynamic stretching: Dynamic stretching involves moving your muscles through a range of motion to loosen them up and prepare them for your workout. Examples include arm swings, leg swings, and lunge walks.

Foam rolling: Foam rolling can help to loosen up tight muscles and increase blood flow, making it an important part of your warm-up routine.

Cool-Down:

Stretching: After your workout, it's important to stretch your muscles to prevent stiffness and injury. Hold each stretch for about 20-30 seconds and focus on breathing deeply.

Yoga: Yoga is a great way to cool down after a workout and stretch your muscles. Incorporating yoga into your cool-down routine can help to improve your flexibility, balance, and focus.

Light cardio: Finish your workout with a few minutes of light cardio exercises, such as walking or light jogging, to help bring your heart rate down and aid in recovery.

By incorporating these warm-up and cool-down techniques into your strength training routine, you can improve your performance and reduce the risk of injury.

Importance of Proper Form

Proper form is crucial when performing dumbbell exercises, as it helps to ensure that you are getting the maximum benefit from your workout while minimizing the risk of injury. Here are some key points to keep in mind when it comes to proper form:

Stand tall: Stand with your feet hip-width apart, your core engaged, and your shoulders back and down. This will help you maintain good posture and stability during your workout.

Engage your core: Engaging your core helps to stabilize your spine and protect your lower back. Focus on contracting your abdominal muscles throughout each exercise.

Keep your shoulders relaxed: Tension in your shoulders can limit your range of motion and lead to injury. Keep your shoulders relaxed and down throughout your workout.

Control the weight: Moving too quickly or using too much weight can increase your risk of injury. Focus on controlling the weight throughout each movement, and avoid using momentum to complete the exercise.

Focus on the muscles you are working: As you perform each exercise, focus on the muscles you are working, and feel the burn in those muscles. This will help you get the most out of your workout.

CHAPTER III: TOTAL BODY WORKOUTS

Upper Body Workouts

Upper body workouts are essential for building strength and toning your arms, chest, back, and shoulders. Here are some of the most effective dumbbell exercises for women:

Dumbbell Shoulder Press

Step-by-step instructions:

1. Stand with your feet shoulder-width apart, holding a dumbbell in each hand at shoulder height.
2. Push the weights overhead, keeping your wrists straight and elbows under the weights.
3. Lower the weights back to your starting position.

Muscle focus: Shoulders

Safety tips: Avoid arching your back and keep your core engaged.

Repetitions and sets: 3 sets of 12-15 reps

Variation: Seated shoulder press or Arnold press

Progression: Increase the weight of the dumbbells.

Dumbbell Flys

Step-by-step instructions:

1. Lie on a flat bench with your feet flat on the floor.
2. Hold a dumbbell in each hand above your chest, palms facing each other.
3. Lower the weights out to the sides, keeping a slight bend in your elbows.
4. Return the weights to the starting position.

Muscle focus: Chest

Safety tips: Avoid arching your back and keep your core engaged.

Repetitions and sets: 3 sets of 12-15 reps

Variation: Incline dumbbell flys or decline dumbbell flys

Progression: Increase the weight of the dumbbells.

Dumbbell Lat Pulldowns

Step-by-step instructions:

1. Stand with your feet shoulder-width apart, holding a dumbbell in each hand.

2. Pull the weights down to your sides, keeping your elbows close to your body.
3. Return the weights to the starting position.

Muscle focus: Lats

Safety tips: Avoid swinging the weights and keep your shoulders relaxed.

Repetitions and sets: 3 sets of 12-15 reps

Variation: Seated lat pulldowns or single arm lat pulldowns

Progression: Increase the weight of the dumbbells.

Dumbbell Bent Over Rows
Step-by-Step Instructions:

1. Start by standing with your feet hip-width apart, holding a dumbbell in each hand.
2. Hinge forward from your hips, keeping your back flat and bend your knees slightly.
3. Your arms should hang down straight, palms facing each other.
4. Exhale and pull the dumbbells up towards your chest, keeping your elbows close to your body.
5. Inhale and lower the dumbbells back to the starting position, keeping your back flat.

Muscle Focus: The bent over row targets the back, shoulders, and biceps.

Safety Tips:

- Make sure your back stays flat throughout the exercise to avoid injury.
- Keep your movements slow and controlled to maintain proper form.
- Avoid arching your back, which can cause injury to the lower back.

Repetitions: 3 sets of 8-12 reps

Variation: Dumbbell One Arm Bent Over Rows

Progression: Increase the weight of the dumbbells.

Dumbbell Chest Press
Step-by-Step Instructions:

1. Start by lying on a flat bench, holding a dumbbell in each hand above your chest, palms facing away from your body.
2. Keep your feet flat on the floor, with your knees bent at 90 degrees.
3. Exhale and press the dumbbells upwards, keeping your elbows tucked in.
4. Inhale and lower the dumbbells back to the starting position.

Muscle Focus: The chest press targets the chest, triceps, and shoulders.

Safety Tips:

- Make sure your back stays flat on the bench throughout the exercise to maintain proper form.
- Avoid locking your elbows at the top of the movement.
- Keep your movements slow and controlled.

Repetitions: 3 sets of 8-12 reps

Variation: Dumbbell Incline Chest Press

Progression: Increase the weight of the dumbbells.

Dumbbell Upright Rows

1. Stand with your feet shoulder-width apart and hold a dumbbell in each hand, with your palms facing your thighs.
2. Keeping your arms straight, lift the dumbbells towards your chest, keeping them close to your body.
3. As you lift the dumbbells, rotate your palms to face your body and continue to lift until the weights reach your chest.
4. Pause at the top of the movement, then slowly lower the weights back to the starting position.

Muscle focus: Shoulders, traps, and upper back.

Safety tips:

- Avoid lifting the weights too high, as this can put stress on your shoulders and lead to injury.
- Keep your movements slow and controlled to reduce the risk of injury.

Repetitions and sets: 3 sets of 10 reps.

Variation: Barbell upright rows, cable face pulls, shoulder press.

Progression: Increase the weight or reps, or add an additional set to increase the intensity of the exercise.

Dumbbell Rear Delt Flys
Step-by-Step Instructions:

1. Start by standing with feet hip-width apart and holding a dumbbell in each hand.
2. Bend forward at the hips until your torso is parallel to the floor.
3. Keep your back straight and abs engaged.
4. With arms straight and hands pointing downwards, lift the dumbbells out to the sides, keeping your elbows slightly bent.
5. Stop when your arms are parallel to the floor.
6. Slowly lower the weights back to the starting position.

Muscle Focus: The primary muscles worked in this exercise are the rear deltoids and the rhomboids.

Safety Tips: To avoid straining your lower back, make sure you have proper form and keep your back straight throughout the exercise.

Repetitions and Sets: Start with 3 sets of 10 repetitions, gradually increasing as you get stronger.

Variation and Progression: To progress, increase the weight of the dumbbells or increase the number of sets and repetitions.

Dumbbell Lateral Raises
Step-by-Step Instructions:

1. Stand with feet hip-width apart and hold a dumbbell in each hand.
2. Keep your arms straight and pointing downwards.
3. Lift the weights out to the sides, keeping your elbows slightly bent.
4. Stop when your arms are parallel to the floor.
5. Slowly lower the weights back to the starting position.

Muscle Focus: The primary muscle worked in this exercise is the lateral deltoid.

Safety Tips: Avoid swinging the weights and keep the movement controlled. Also, avoid locking your elbows to prevent injury.

Repetitions and Sets: Start with 3 sets of 10 repetitions, gradually increasing as you get stronger.

Variation and Progression: To progress, increase the weight of the dumbbells or increase the number of sets and repetitions.

Dumbbell Front Delt Raises

Step-by-Step Instructions:

1. Stand with feet hip-width apart and hold a dumbbell in each hand.
2. Keep your arms straight and pointing downwards.
3. Lift the weights straight up in front of your body, keeping your elbows slightly bent.
4. Stop when your arms are parallel to the floor.
5. Slowly lower the weights back to the starting position.

Muscle Focus: The primary muscle worked in this exercise is the front deltoid.

Safety Tips: Avoid swinging the weights and keep the movement controlled. Also, avoid locking your elbows to prevent injury.

Repetitions and Sets: Start with 3 sets of 10 repetitions, gradually increasing as you get stronger.

Variation and Progression: To progress, increase the weight of the dumbbells or increase the number of sets and repetitions.

Dumbbell Overhead Tricep Extensions

1. Begin by standing up straight with your feet hip-width apart and holding a pair of dumbbells over your head with your palms facing each other.
2. Lower the dumbbells behind your head by bending at the elbows, keeping your upper arms close to your head and your elbows pointing forward.
3. Exhale and extend your arms back to the starting position.
4. Repeat for 10-12 repetitions, completing 3 sets.

Muscle focus: Triceps, Shoulders

Safety tips:

- Keep your back straight throughout the exercise to avoid injury to your lower back.
- Avoid locking your elbows at the top of the movement.

Variation: This exercise can also be performed seated or on a bench to isolate the triceps.

Progression: As you get stronger, increase the weight of the dumbbells or increase the number of sets.

Lower Body Workouts

Dumbbell Squats

1. Start with feet shoulder-width apart, holding dumbbells in front of the chest with both hands.
2. Slowly lower your body into a squatting position while keeping the weight of your body on your heels.
3. Push back up to the starting position, exhaling as you stand.

Focus: Quads, Glutes, Hamstrings

Safety Tips: Keep your knees behind your toes, avoid arching your lower back.

Repetitions: 3 sets of 12-15 reps

Variation: Goblet Squats, Sumo Squats, Plié Squats

Progression: Increase weight of dumbbells, add one more set or reps

Dumbbell Lunges

1. Stand with feet hip-width apart, holding dumbbells in each hand.
2. Take a large step forward with one foot and lower your body towards the ground until both legs are bent at a 90-degree angle.
3. Push back up to the starting position, bringing the other foot forward to repeat the movement.

Focus: Quads, Glutes, Hamstrings

Safety Tips: Keep the front knee behind the toes, avoid leaning forward.

Repetitions: 3 sets of 12-15 reps per leg

Variation: Walking Lunges, Reverse Lunges, Side Lunges

Progression: Increase weight of dumbbells, add one more set or reps

Dumbbell Sumo Squats

1. Stand with your feet wider than shoulder-width apart, toes pointed outwards.
2. Hold the dumbbells at shoulder height, palms facing inwards.
3. Slowly lower your body down towards the ground, keeping your back straight and your core engaged.
4. Push through your heels to return to the starting position.

Repeat 8-12 times for 3 sets.

Muscle Focus: Glutes, Hamstrings, Quadriceps

Safety Tips:

- Keep your back straight and core engaged throughout the exercise.
- Avoid rounding your back or arching too far backwards.

Variation: You can also perform a sumo squat with one dumbbell, holding it in front of your chest.

Progression: Increase the weight of the dumbbells, or perform a sumo squat with a barbell.

Dumbbell Hamstring Curls
1. Lie face down on a flat surface, with your legs extended.
2. Hold the dumbbells with your feet.
3. Bend your knees, lifting the weights towards your butt.
4. Lower the weights back down to the starting position.
5. Repeat 8-12 times for 3 sets.

Muscle Focus: Hamstrings

Safety Tips:

- Keep your hips steady and avoid lifting them off the ground.
- Use a mat for cushioning if needed.

Variation: You can also perform the exercise with a stability ball.

Progression: Increase the weight of the dumbbells.

Dumbbell Step-Ups
1. Stand in front of a bench or box, with a dumbbell in each hand.

2. Step onto the bench with your right foot, pressing through the heel to stand tall.
3. Step back down with your right foot, followed by your left.
4. Repeat on the other side.

Repeat 8-12 times for 3 sets.

Muscle Focus: Quadriceps, Glutes, Hamstrings

Safety Tips:

- Make sure the bench or box is stable and secure.
- Avoid twisting your hips or knees.

Variation: You can perform the exercise with one dumbbell, or with a barbell.

Progression: Increase the height of the bench or box.

Dumbbell Calf Raises
Step-by-Step Instructions:

1. Start by standing with your feet shoulder-width apart, holding a dumbbell in each hand by your sides.
2. Rise up onto your toes, lifting the weights as high as you can.
3. Pause for a moment at the top, then slowly lower back down to the starting position.

Muscle Focus: The primary muscles worked in this exercise are the calf muscles.

Safety Tips: Make sure to keep your knees slightly bent throughout the exercise to avoid putting too much pressure on your knee joints.

Repetitions and Sets: Start with 3 sets of 10-12 reps and gradually increase as you become stronger.

Variation and Progression: To make the exercise more challenging, you can stand on a raised platform such as a step or plate.

Dumbbell Side Lunges
Step-by-Step Instructions:

1. Start by standing with your feet shoulder-width apart, holding a dumbbell in each hand at your sides.
2. Take a step to the side, lowering your body down as far as you can while keeping your back straight.
3. Push back up to the starting position, then repeat on the other side.

Muscle Focus: The primary muscles worked in this exercise are the quadriceps, hamstrings, and glutes.

Safety Tips: Make sure to keep your front knee behind your front toes to avoid putting too much pressure on your knee joint.

Repetitions and Sets: Start with 3 sets of 10-12 reps on each side and gradually increase as you become stronger.

Variation and Progression: To make the exercise more challenging, you can hold heavier dumbbells or perform the exercise on an unstable surface such as a balance ball.

Dumbbell Box Jumps
Step-by-Step Instructions:

1. Start by standing in front of a sturdy box or platform, holding a dumbbell in each hand at your sides.
2. Explosively jump up onto the box, landing with both feet on the surface.
3. Step back down to the starting position and repeat.

Muscle Focus: The primary muscles worked in this exercise are the quadriceps, hamstrings, and glutes.

Safety Tips: Make sure to warm up thoroughly before attempting this exercise, and choose a box height that is appropriate for your current level of fitness.

Repetitions and Sets: Start with 3 sets of 8-10 reps and gradually increase as you become stronger.

Variation and Progression: To make the exercise more challenging, you can hold heavier dumbbells or increase the height of the box.

Dumbbell Box Squats

Step-by-step instructions:

1. Stand with your feet hip-width apart and place a low box or bench behind you.
2. Hold a dumbbell in each hand and lower down into a squat, keeping your chest up and your weight in your heels.
3. Touch your buttocks to the box, pause for a second, then stand back up, squeezing your glutes at the top.

Muscle Focus: Glutes, hamstrings, quadriceps

Safety Tips:

- Make sure to keep your weight in your heels throughout the exercise
- Keep your chest up and avoid hunching over
- Avoid letting your knees extend past your toes

Repetitions and Sets: Start with 2-3 sets of 10-12 repetitions

Variation and Progression:

- To increase difficulty, increase the weight of your dumbbells
- To make the exercise easier, decrease the weight of your dumbbells or perform the exercise without weights

Dumbbell Plié Squats

1. Start by standing with your feet slightly wider than hip-width apart, with your toes turned out.
2. Hold a dumbbell in each hand and bring them up to your shoulders.
3. Begin the squat by lowering your hips down and back as if you are sitting back into a chair.
4. Keep your knees turned out and your weight in your heels.
5. Go as low as you can while keeping your heels on the ground.
6. Pause at the bottom of the squat and then press through your heels to stand back up.
7. Repeat the movement for 8-12 repetitions and complete 3 sets.

Muscle Focus: Glutes, hamstrings, and quadriceps.

Safety Tips: Keep your knees turned out and avoid letting them cave in. Keep your back straight and avoid hunching forward.

Variation: To increase the challenge, try doing plié squats on one leg at a time.

Progression: To progress this exercise, you can use heavier dumbbells or try doing plyometric plié squats, jumping as you stand back up from the squat.

Dumbbell Fire Hydrants

1. Start on all fours with a dumbbell in each hand.
2. Keep your left knee bent and your left foot flat on the ground.
3. Lift your right leg out to the side, keeping your knee bent and your foot flexed.
4. Hold the position for a count of two and then return your leg to the starting position.
5. Repeat the movement for 8-12 repetitions on each side and complete 3 sets.

Muscle Focus: Glutes and hips.

Safety Tips: Keep your back straight and avoid arching your back. Keep your movements controlled and slow.

Variation: To increase the challenge, try lifting your leg higher and holding the position for a longer count.

Progression: To progress this exercise, you can use heavier dumbbells or try adding in a small pulse at the top of the movement.

Core Workouts

Dumbbell Side Plank

1. Begin by lying on your side with your legs extended and your elbow bent directly beneath your shoulder.
2. Hold a dumbbell in your top hand, and extend your arm straight up towards the ceiling.
3. Keep your body in a straight line, engage your core and hold the position for a set amount of time.

Muscle focus: Obliques, transverse abdominis, rectus abdominis, gluteus medius

Safety tips: Keep your body in a straight line, and avoid sinking towards the floor.

Repetitions: Start with holding the position for 30 seconds, and gradually increase as you build strength.

Sets: 3-4 sets on each side

Variation: You can also perform this exercise without a dumbbell or with a heavier weight for added resistance.

Progression: Increase the time that you hold the position, or add an additional set.

Dumbbell Sit-Ups

1. Begin by lying on your back with your knees bent and feet flat on the floor.
2. Hold a dumbbell in both hands, with your arms extended straight above your head.
3. Sit up, lifting the dumbbell towards your knees.
4. Keep your back straight and core engaged throughout the movement.

Muscle focus: Rectus abdominis, obliques, hip flexors

Safety tips: Keep your neck relaxed and avoid pulling on your head or neck. Keep your back straight and avoid arching your back.

Repetitions: Start with 10-15 repetitions, and gradually increase as you build strength.

Sets: 3-4 sets

Variation: You can also perform this exercise with a medicine ball or a kettlebell for added resistance.

Progression: Increase the weight of the dumbbell or add additional repetitions.

Dumbbell Leg Raises
Step-by-Step Instructions:

1. Lie down on your back with your feet together and your arms extended straight along your sides.
2. Hold a dumbbell in each hand and keep your palms facing down.
3. Keep your feet together and raise them off the ground until your legs are perpendicular to your body.
4. Lower your legs back to the starting position.
5. Repeat for the desired number of repetitions.

Muscle Focus: The main focus of this exercise is on the rectus abdominis, the oblique muscles and the hip flexors.

Safety Tips:

- Keep your lower back pressed into the ground throughout the exercise.
- Do not swing your legs while performing the movement.
- Do not arch your back during the exercise.

Repetitions and Sets: Begin with 2-3 sets of 10-15 repetitions, gradually increasing the number of sets and reps as you progress.

Variation: You can make the exercise more challenging by holding a weight plate or a medicine ball between your feet.

Progression: To progress, you can raise both legs and your arms at the same time, keeping the weight in your hands.

Dumbbell Plank Holds

1. Begin in a plank position, with hands resting on the dumbbells.
2. Keep your core tight and maintain proper form by keeping your back straight and your head in line with your spine.
3. Hold this position for 30-60 seconds, or as long as you can maintain proper form.
4. Repeat for 3-5 sets.

Muscle Focus: Core, shoulders, and triceps.

Safety Tips: Make sure to keep your neck and spine in alignment, and do not let your hips drop or raise too high.

Repetitions: Hold for 30-60 seconds per set.

Sets: 3-5 sets.

Variation: Increase the duration of the hold, or add a side plank for added challenge.

Progression: Increase the weight of the dumbbells for added resistance.

Dumbbell Scissor Kicks

1. Lie flat on your back, with dumbbells in your hands, arms extended straight overhead.

2. Lift your legs off the ground and alternate kicking one leg towards your chest while keeping the other leg straight.
3. Repeat for 10-15 reps per side.
4. Repeat for 3-5 sets.

Muscle Focus: Core, lower abs.

Safety Tips: Keep your back flat against the ground and avoid lifting your neck or shoulders.

Repetitions: 10-15 reps per side.

Sets: 3-5 sets.

Variation: Add a twist for an added challenge.

Progression: Increase the weight of the dumbbells for added resistance.

Dumbbell Woodchoppers
1. Stand with feet shoulder-width apart, holding a dumbbell with both hands.
2. Raise the dumbbell overhead, twisting your torso and bringing the dumbbell down to the opposite hip.
3. Repeat for 10-15 reps per side.
4. Repeat for 3-5 sets.

Muscle Focus: Core, obliques, and shoulders.

Safety Tips: Keep your neck and spine in alignment and use controlled movements.

Repetitions: 10-15 reps per side.

Sets: 3-5 sets.

Variation: Add a squat for an added challenge.

Progression: Increase the weight of the dumbbells for added resistance.

Dumbbell Leg Lifts
Step-by-step instructions:

1. Lie on your back with your arms at your sides and hold a dumbbell in each hand.
2. Keeping your legs straight, lift both legs up towards the ceiling until they form a 90-degree angle with your torso.
3. Lower your legs back down, but don't let them touch the ground.
4. Repeat for a set amount of repetitions.

Muscle focus: Lower abs, hips, and glutes

Safety tips:

- Keep your neck relaxed and don't use your arms to lift your legs.

- Also, keep your legs straight and don't let them touch the ground between reps.

Repetitions and sets: Begin with 3 sets of 10 repetitions, and progress as you feel comfortable.

Variation: Try lifting one leg at a time for a single-leg variation.

Progression: Hold the dumbbells closer to your feet or use heavier dumbbells.

Dumbbell Bicycles
Step-by-step instructions:

1. Start by lying flat on your back with your hands behind your head.
2. Hold a dumbbell in each hand and extend your arms toward the ceiling.
3. Bring your right knee toward your chest while simultaneously lifting your torso and left knee off the ground.
4. Reach your left elbow towards your right knee as you lower it back to the starting position.
5. Repeat the movement on the opposite side, bringing your left knee toward your chest while simultaneously lifting your torso and right knee off the ground.
6. Reach your right elbow towards your left knee.

Continue alternating between sides for the desired number of repetitions.

Muscle Focus: The Dumbbell Bicycles primarily work the abs and obliques, but also engage the hip flexors and lower back muscles.

Safety Tips:

- Avoid pulling on your neck or head with your hands. Keep your hands relaxed behind your head.
- Keep your low back pressed into the floor to avoid overarch.
- If you experience discomfort in your lower back, you can place a small pillow under your lumbar spine.

Repetitions and Sets:

- Begin with 2-3 sets of 8-12 repetitions on each side.
- As you progress, aim to increase the number of repetitions and sets.

Variation and Progression:

- To increase the intensity, you can use heavier dumbbells or add an exercise ball to the mix.
- You can also perform the exercise with one leg lifted off the ground for an added challenge.

Dumbbell Reverse Sit-Ups

Step-by-step instructions:

1. Start by lying flat on your back with your legs extended and your arms overhead holding a dumbbell in each hand.
2. Sit up and reach towards your toes, lifting the dumbbells towards your feet.
3. Lower back down to the starting position.
4. Repeat the movement for the desired number of repetitions.

Muscle Focus: The Dumbbell Reverse Sit-Ups primarily target the rectus abdominis (six-pack muscle), but also engage the obliques, hip flexors, and lower back muscles.

Safety Tips:

- Keep your low back pressed into the floor to avoid overarch.
- Avoid pulling on your neck or head with your hands. Keep your hands relaxed and let the dumbbells guide the movement.
- If you experience discomfort in your lower back, you can place a small pillow under your lumbar spine.

Repetitions and Sets:

- Begin with 2-3 sets of 8-12 repetitions.
- As you progress, aim to increase the number of repetitions and sets.

Variation and Progression:

- To increase the intensity, you can use heavier dumbbells.
- You can also perform the exercise with one leg lifted off the ground for an added challenge.

Dumbbell Toe Touches

Step-by-Step Instructions:

1. Start by lying flat on your back on a mat or soft surface, with your knees bent and feet flat on the floor.
2. Hold a dumbbell in each hand and extend your arms straight up towards the ceiling.
3. Keeping your arms extended, reach for your left toes with your left hand.
4. Slowly return to the starting position and repeat the same motion on the other side, reaching for your right toes with your right hand.
5. Repeat for desired repetitions.

Muscle Focus: This exercise focuses on the rectus abdominis, obliques, and lower back muscles.

Safety Tips:

- Keep your neck relaxed and maintain proper alignment of your spine throughout the movement.

- Avoid arching your back or lifting your shoulder blades off the ground.

Repetitions and Sets: Begin with 2-3 sets of 8-12 repetitions on each side, gradually increasing as you get stronger.

Variation and Progression: To increase the difficulty, you can straighten your legs, hold heavier dumbbells, or add a twist to the movement.

Dumbbell Spiderman Plank

Step-by-Step Instructions:

1. Start in a high plank position, with your hands holding dumbbells on the floor directly under your shoulders.
2. As you exhale, bring your right knee towards your right elbow.
3. Return to the starting position and repeat on the other side, bringing your left knee towards your left elbow.
4. Repeat for desired repetitions.

Muscle Focus: This exercise focuses on the rectus abdominis, obliques, hip flexors, and lower back muscles.

Safety Tips:

- Keep your back straight and maintain proper alignment of your spine throughout the movement.
- Avoid letting your hips sag or twisting too far to one side.

Repetitions and Sets: Begin with 2-3 sets of 8-12 repetitions on each side, gradually increasing as you get stronger.

Variation and Progression: To increase the difficulty, you can hold heavier dumbbells, pause in the middle of the movement, or extend your legs straight instead of keeping them bent.

Full-Body Workouts

Dumbbell Squat and Press
Step-by-Step Instructions:

1. Start with feet shoulder-width apart and hold a dumbbell in each hand.
2. Lower down into a squat position, making sure your knees are aligned with your toes and your weight is in your heels.
3. Push back up to standing position and press the dumbbells overhead.
4. Repeat the movement for the desired number of repetitions.

Muscle Focus: Legs, glutes, and shoulders

Safety Tips:

- Keep your core engaged and maintain proper form throughout the movement.
- Avoid rounding your back or allowing your knees to cave inwards.

Repetitions and Sets: 3 sets of 10-15 repetitions

Variation and Progression: Increase the weight of the dumbbells or add an explosive jump into the press movement for an added challenge.

Dumbbell Lunges with Bicep Curls
Step-by-Step Instructions:

1. Stand with your feet shoulder-width apart, holding a dumbbell in each hand.
2. Step forward with one foot and lower down into a lunge position, keeping your front knee aligned with your ankle.
3. Push back up to standing position and curl the dumbbells towards your shoulders.
4. Repeat the movement with the other leg and continue alternating for the desired number of repetitions.

Muscle Focus: Legs, glutes, biceps, and core

Safety Tips: Keep your core engaged and maintain proper form throughout the movement. Avoid letting your front knee extend past your toes.

Repetitions and Sets: 3 sets of 10-15 repetitions on each leg

Variation and Progression: Increase the weight of the dumbbells or add a lunge jump for an added challenge.

Dumbbell Plank to Push-Up
Step-by-Step instructions:

1. Begin in a plank position with dumbbells in each hand and feet shoulder-width apart.
2. Keep your core tight and maintain a straight line from head to heels.
3. Lower yourself down until your chest almost touches the ground and push back up, keeping your elbow close to your body.
4. Repeat for the desired number of repetitions.

Muscle Focus: Core, chest, triceps, and shoulders.

Safety Tips:

- Make sure to maintain proper form throughout the exercise to avoid injury.
- Keep your neck in line with your spine and avoid arching or rounding your back.

Repetitions and Sets: Start with 3 sets of 8-12 repetitions and gradually increase as you get stronger.

Variation: To make the exercise easier, you can perform the push-ups on your knees instead of your toes. To make it harder, you can increase the weight of the dumbbells.

Progression: To progress, you can try performing the push-up on a stability ball or adding a medicine ball for added resistance.

Dumbbell Russian Twists
Step-by-Step instructions:

1. Sit on the ground with your knees bent and feet flat on the floor.
2. Hold a dumbbell with both hands and lean back slightly, keeping your core engaged.
3. Twist your torso to the left, then to the right, keeping the dumbbell close to your body.
4. Repeat for the desired number of repetitions.

Muscle Focus: Obliques, abs, and lower back.

Safety Tips:

- Make sure to maintain proper form throughout the exercise to avoid injury.
- Keep your neck in line with your spine and avoid arching or rounding your back.

Repetitions and Sets: Start with 3 sets of 12-15 repetitions on each side and gradually increase as you get stronger.

Variation:

- To make the exercise easier, you can perform the exercise without a dumbbell or with a lighter weight.
- To make it harder, you can increase the weight of the dumbbell or perform the exercise on a stability ball.

Progression: To progress, you can try adding a pulse or a hold at the end of each repetition for added resistance.

Dumbbell Clean and Jerk

Step-by-step instructions:

1. Stand with your feet shoulder-width apart, holding a dumbbell in each hand.
2. Bend at the knees, keeping your back straight, and lower the dumbbells to your thighs.
3. With a quick explosive movement, push your legs up and stand up, lifting the dumbbells above your head.
4. Dip slightly at the knees and then extend your arms, pressing the dumbbells overhead.
5. Lower the dumbbells to your thighs, bending at the knees and keeping your back straight.

Muscle focus: This exercise works your legs, back, and shoulders.

Safety tips:

- Keep your back straight throughout the movement to avoid injury.
- Make sure to use proper form when lifting the dumbbells overhead.
- If you're new to the exercise, start with lighter weights and gradually increase the weight as you get stronger.

Repetitions and sets: Start with 3 sets of 8 reps, and gradually increase the weight and reps as you get stronger.

Variation: You can perform this exercise with one dumbbell at a time, alternating between sides.

Progression: As you get stronger, you can increase the weight of the dumbbells and perform more reps and sets.

Dumbbell Bulgarian Split Squats
Step-by-step instructions:

1. Stand with your feet hip-width apart, holding a dumbbell in each hand.
2. Step your right foot behind you, placing it on a bench or step.
3. Bend your left knee and lower your body until your left knee is bent to a 90-degree angle.
4. Push yourself back up, straightening your left leg.
5. Repeat for the desired number of reps and then switch sides.

Muscle focus: This exercise works your glutes, hamstrings, and quads.

Safety tips:

- Make sure to keep your core engaged and your back straight throughout the movement.
- Keep your front knee aligned with your ankle to avoid knee injury.
- Make sure the bench or step is sturdy and secure.

Repetitions and sets: Start with 3 sets of 8 reps on each side, and gradually increase the reps and sets as you get stronger.

Variation: You can perform this exercise without weights, using just your body weight for resistance.

Progression: As you get stronger, you can increase the weight of the dumbbells and perform more reps and sets.

Dumbbell Reverse Flys
Step-by-step instructions:

1. Start by standing with your feet shoulder-width apart, holding a pair of dumbbells at hip height.
2. Hinge forward from the hips and keep your back straight, so that your torso is parallel to the floor.
3. From this position, lift the dumbbells away from your body, keeping your arms straight, until they are level with your shoulders.

4. Pause briefly, then slowly lower the weights back to the starting position.

Muscle focus: The reverse fly primarily targets the upper back, shoulder and shoulder blade muscles (trapezius, rhomboids, and rotator cuff).

Safety tips: Keep your back straight and avoid rounding your shoulders. It is important to maintain proper form to avoid injury to your shoulders or back.

Repetitions and sets: Start with 2-3 sets of 8-12 repetitions, gradually increasing the number of sets and reps as you get stronger.

Variation and progression: To increase the intensity of the exercise, increase the weight of the dumbbells or add a small balance challenge, such as standing on a stability ball.

Dumbbell Mountain Climbers
Step-by-Step Instructions:

1. Start in a push-up position with a dumbbell in each hand.
2. Bring one knee up towards your chest, keeping the other leg straight.
3. Return to the starting position and repeat with the other leg.

Muscle Focus: Abs, Obliques, Quadriceps, and Hamstrings.

Safety Tips:

- Keep your core engaged and avoid sagging your lower back.
- Keep your elbows close to your body to avoid strain on your shoulders.
- Avoid any bouncing or jerking movements.

Repetitions: 20-25 for 3 sets.

Variation and Progression:

- Increase the speed and intensity of the movement.
- Add a jump when bringing your knee up to make the exercise more challenging.

Dumbbell Thruster

Step-by-Step Instructions:

1. Stand with your feet hip-width apart, holding a pair of dumbbells at shoulder height.
2. Lower your hips down into a squat, keeping your chest up and your weight in your heels.
3. Push through your heels to stand up, pressing the dumbbells overhead.
4. Lower the weights back to shoulder height, and repeat the movement for your desired number of repetitions.

Muscle Focus: This full-body workout primarily focuses on the legs, glutes, and shoulders.

Safety Tips:

- Make sure to keep your chest up and your weight in your heels as you squat.
- Use proper form when pressing the weights overhead, keeping your arms straight and your shoulders down.
- Start with lighter weights and gradually increase as you build strength and confidence.

Repetitions and Sets: Start with 2-3 sets of 8-12 repetitions, and gradually increase as you build strength and confidence.

Variation: You can also perform this exercise using a single dumbbell or kettlebell for added challenge.

Progression: To progress, increase the weight of the dumbbells or add additional sets and reps.

Dumbbell Squat Jumps
Step-by-Step Instructions:

1. Stand with your feet hip-width apart, holding a pair of dumbbells at your sides.
2. Lower your hips down into a squat, keeping your chest up and your weight in your heels.
3. Push through your heels to jump up, landing softly back in the squat position.

4. Repeat the movement for your desired number of repetitions.

Muscle Focus: This full-body workout primarily focuses on the legs, glutes, and core.

Safety Tips:

- Make sure to use proper form as you squat and jump, keeping your chest up and your weight in your heels.
- Start with lighter weights and gradually increase as you build strength and confidence.
- Warm up thoroughly before performing this exercise to avoid injury.

Repetitions and Sets: Start with 2-3 sets of 8-12 repetitions, and gradually increase as you build strength and confidence.

Variation: You can also perform this exercise without weights for added challenge.

Progression: To progress, increase the weight of the dumbbells or add additional sets and reps.

CHAPTER IV: TARGETED WORKOUTS

Arms and Shoulders

Dumbbell Bicep Curls
Step-by-Step Instructions:

1. Stand with your feet shoulder-width apart and your knees slightly bent.
2. Hold the dumbbells in each hand with an underhand grip.
3. Keep your elbows close to your sides and slowly curl the weights towards your shoulders.
4. Hold for a second at the top of the movement before lowering back to the starting position.

Muscle Focus: Biceps

Safety Tips:

- Keep your elbows close to your sides to avoid putting unnecessary strain on your shoulders.
- Don't swing the weights or use momentum to complete the reps.

- Make sure to warm up before starting the exercise.

Repetitions and Sets: 3 sets of 10-12 reps

Variation and Progression: To increase the difficulty, use heavier weights or complete the exercise in a slow and controlled manner.

Dumbbell Tricep Extensions
Step-by-Step Instructions:

1. Stand with your feet shoulder-width apart and your knees slightly bent.
2. Hold a dumbbell in both hands above your head with your palms facing each other.
3. Lower the weight behind your head, keeping your elbows close to your ears.
4. Push the weight back up to the starting position.

Muscle Focus: Triceps

Safety Tips:

- Make sure to warm up before starting the exercise.
- Don't arch your back or use momentum to complete the reps.
- Keep your elbows close to your ears to avoid injury.

Repetitions and Sets: 3 sets of 10-12 reps

Variation and Progression: To increase the difficulty, use heavier weights or complete the exercise in a slow and controlled manner.

Dumbbell Hammer Curls

Step-by-Step Instructions:

1. Stand with your feet shoulder-width apart and your knees slightly bent.
2. Hold the dumbbells in each hand with a neutral grip (palms facing each other).
3. Keep your elbows close to your sides and slowly curl the weights towards your shoulders.
4. Hold for a second at the top of the movement before lowering back to the starting position.

Muscle Focus: Biceps and Forearms

Safety Tips:

- Make sure to warm up before starting the exercise.
- Don't swing the weights or use momentum to complete the reps.
- Keep your elbows close to your sides to avoid putting unnecessary strain on your shoulders.

Repetitions and Sets: 3 sets of 10-12 reps

Variation and Progression: To increase the difficulty, use heavy weights or complete the exercise in a slow and controlled manner.

Dumbbell Shrugs

Step-by-Step Instructions:

1. Stand with your feet shoulder-width apart and hold a pair of dumbbells at your sides.
2. Keeping your arms straight, lift the dumbbells towards your shoulders while keeping your shoulders relaxed.
3. Hold for a second and then lower the weights back down.

Muscle Focus: Traps and Upper Back

Safety Tips:

- Avoid rolling your shoulders or bending your arms during the exercise.
- Keep your core engaged and maintain a neutral spine throughout the movement.

Repetitions and Sets: Start with 3 sets of 12-15 reps and gradually increase as you get stronger.

Variation and Progression: You can add weight as you get stronger, or perform the shrugs with a barbell instead of dumbbells.

Dumbbell Pullovers

Step-by-Step Instructions:

1. Lie flat on a bench or mat with a dumbbell held above your chest with both hands.
2. Lower the weight behind your head, keeping your arms straight and engaging your back muscles.
3. Return the weight back to the starting position.

Muscle Focus: Chest, Back, and Triceps

Safety Tips:

- Keep your neck and spine aligned throughout the exercise.
- Do not arch your back during the movement.

Repetitions and Sets: Start with 3 sets of 8-10 reps and gradually increase as you get stronger.

Variation and Progression: You can perform the exercise with a barbell or change the angle of the bench for a greater challenge.

Dumbbell Concentration Curls

Step-by-Step Instructions:

1. Sit on a bench or chair with a dumbbell in one hand.
2. Plant your elbow on the inside of your thigh, and curl the weight towards your shoulder.

3. Lower the weight back down to the starting position.

Muscle Focus: Biceps

Safety Tips:

- Keep your upper arm stationary and avoid swinging the weight during the exercise.
- Engage your core for stability.

Repetitions and Sets: Start with 3 sets of 8-10 reps per arm and gradually increase as you get stronger.

Variation and Progression: You can perform the exercise with a barbell or change the angle of your wrist for a different challenge.

Dumbbell Close Grip Bench Press
Step-by-step instructions:

1. Lie flat on a weight bench with a dumbbell in each hand.
2. Keep your feet firmly on the floor and your back flat against the bench.
3. With your palms facing each other, position the dumbbells just outside of your chest.
4. Lower the dumbbells slowly to your chest, then press them back up to the starting position.
5. Repeat for the desired number of repetitions and sets.

Muscle focus: triceps, chest, shoulders

Safety tips:

- Keep your back flat against the bench and your feet firmly on the floor for stability.
- Do not lower the dumbbells too far, as this can strain your elbow and shoulder joints.
- Warm up with lighter weights before increasing the weight.

Repetitions and sets: 3 sets of 8-12 repetitions

Progression:

- Increase weight
- Increase repetitions or sets
- Change the angle of the bench

Dumbbell Alternating Curls

Step-by-step instructions:

1. Stand with your feet shoulder-width apart and hold a dumbbell in each hand.
2. Keep your elbows close to your sides and your palms facing forward.
3. Curl one arm up to your shoulder, then lower it back down.
4. Repeat with the other arm.
5. Alternate arms for the desired number of repetitions and sets.

Muscle focus: biceps

Safety tips:

- Keep your back straight and avoid swinging your body to help lift the weights.
- Do not overarch your back or let your elbows flare out.
- Warm up with lighter weights before increasing the weight.

Repetitions and sets: 3 sets of 8-12 repetitions

Variation:

- Standing Dumbbell Hammer Curls
- Seated Dumbbell Alternating Curls

Progression:

- Increase weight
- Increase repetitions or sets
- Change grip position (narrow or wide)

Dumbbell Skull Crushers

Step-by-step instructions:

1. Lie flat on a weight bench with a dumbbell in each hand.
2. Keep your feet firmly on the floor and your back flat against the bench.
3. With your palms facing each other, position the dumbbells above your head.

4. Lower the dumbbells slowly towards your temples, then press them back up to the starting position.
5. Repeat for the desired number of repetitions and sets.

Muscle focus: triceps, chest, shoulders

Safety tips:

- Keep your back flat against the bench and your feet firmly on the floor for stability.
- Do not lower the dumbbells too far, as this can strain your elbow and shoulder joints.
- Warm up with lighter weights before increasing the weight.

Repetitions and sets: 3 sets of 8-12 repetitions

Variation:

- Close Grip Dumbbell Bench Press
- Decline Dumbbell Skull Crushers

Progression:

- Increase weight
- Increase repetitions or sets
- Change grip position (narrow or wide)

Chest and Back

Dumbbell Bench Press

Step-by-Step Instructions:

1. Lie down on a flat bench with your feet firmly planted on the ground.
2. Hold a dumbbell in each hand and extend your arms above your chest, with your palms facing forward.
3. Lower the dumbbells slowly to the sides of your chest, then press them back up to the starting position.

Muscle Focus: Chest, Triceps, and Shoulders

Safety Tips:

- Make sure to keep your feet firmly planted on the ground and your back flat against the bench.
- Use a spotter or a lighter weight if needed.

Repetitions and Sets: 3 sets of 8-12 reps

Variation and Progression: Increase the weight of the dumbbells as you get stronger.

Dumbbell Pullover

Step-by-Step Instructions:

1. Lie down on a flat bench with your head and shoulders hanging off the edge.
2. Hold a dumbbell with both hands and extend your arms above your chest.
3. Lower the dumbbell behind your head, keeping your arms slightly bent, then bring it back up to the starting position.

Muscle Focus: Chest and Lats

Safety Tips:

- Keep your back flat against the bench and do not overstretch your arms.
- Use a spotter or a lighter weight if needed.

Repetitions and Sets: 3 sets of 8-12 reps

Variation and Progression: Increase the weight of the dumbbell as you get stronger.

Dumbbell Row
Step-by-Step Instructions:

1. Stand with your feet shoulder-width apart, holding a dumbbell in each hand.
2. Bend at the waist, keeping your back straight, and let the dumbbells hang down.
3. Pull the dumbbells up towards your chest, then lower them back down to the starting position.

Muscle Focus: Back and Biceps

Safety Tips:

- Keep your back straight and do not round your shoulders.
- Use a lighter weight if needed.

Repetitions and Sets: 3 sets of 8-12 reps

Variation and Progression: Increase the weight of the dumbbells as you get stronger.

Dumbbell Pull-Up

Step-by-Step instructions:

1. Stand facing a horizontal bar, grasp the bar with an overhand grip and hands slightly wider than shoulder-width apart.
2. Hang from the bar, keeping your body straight and core engaged.
3. Pull your body up towards the bar, keeping your chin above the bar.
4. Lower your body back down to the starting position, controlling the movement throughout.

Muscle Focus: The latissimus dorsi, rhomboids, biceps, and forearms.

Safety Tips: Make sure to keep your body straight and avoid swinging or using momentum to complete the exercise.

Repetitions and Sets: 3 sets of 8-12 reps.

Variation and Progression:

- To increase the difficulty of the exercise, add weight using a weight belt or resistance band.
- To switch up the exercise, try using a chin-up grip or using rings or TRX straps.

Dumbbell Chest Fly

Step-by-step instructions:

- Start lying flat on a weight bench with your feet firmly planted on the ground.
- Hold a pair of dumbbells above your chest, arms straight and palms facing each other.
- Lower the weights out to the sides, keeping your arms slightly bent.
- Stop when you feel a stretch in your chest, then squeeze your chest and return to the starting position.

Muscle focus: Chest

Safety tips:

- Make sure to keep your arms slightly bent to avoid putting too much pressure on your elbow joints.
- Keep your neck relaxed and avoid arching your back.

Repetitions and sets: 3 sets of 12 repetitions

Variation: You can try this exercise on a stability ball for added challenge.

Progression: Increase the weight of the dumbbells as you become stronger.

Dumbbell Pulling Kneeling Rows
Step-by-step instructions:

1. Kneel on a mat with your knees hip-width apart and your back straight.
2. Hold a pair of dumbbells and lean forward, keeping your back straight.
3. Pull the weights towards your chest, squeezing your shoulder blades together.
4. Lower the weights back to the starting position.

Muscle focus: Back, biceps, and shoulders

Safety tips:

- Keep your back straight and avoid rounding your spine.
- Use a lighter weight if you feel any discomfort in your lower back.

Repetitions and sets: 3 sets of 12 repetitions

Variation: You can try this exercise with a single dumbbell to work each arm individually.

Progression: Increase the weight of the weights as you become stronger.

Dumbbell Seated Rows

Step-by-step instructions:

1. Sit on a weight bench with your feet firmly planted on the ground.
2. Hold a pair of dumbbells at arm's length and lean forward, keeping your back straight.
3. Pull the weights towards your chest, squeezing your shoulder blades together.
4. Lower the weights back to the starting position.

Muscle focus: Back, biceps, and shoulders

Safety tips:

- Keep your back straight and avoid rounding your spine.
- Use a lighter weight if you feel any discomfort in your lower back.

Repetitions and sets: 3 sets of 12 repetitions

Variation: You can try this exercise with a single dumbbell to work each arm individually.

Progression: Increase the weight of the weights as you become stronger.

Dumbbell Deadlifts

Step-by-step instructions:

1. Stand with your feet shoulder-width apart, holding a pair of dumbbells in front of your thighs with your palms facing your legs.
2. Keep your knees slightly bent and your back straight. Hinge at your hips and bend forward to lower the dumbbells to the floor, keeping the weights close to your legs.
3. Drive your hips forward to stand back up to the starting position.

Muscle focus: Hamstrings, glutes, lower back, and forearms

Safety tips: Keep your back straight, avoid rounding your back and keep your knees slightly bent throughout the exercise.

Repetitions and sets: 3 sets of 8-12 repetitions, with a weight that allows you to complete all reps with good form.

Variation: You can also perform Romanian deadlifts, single-leg deadlifts, or sumo deadlifts with dumbbells.

Progression: Increase the weight of the dumbbells or the number of repetitions as you progress.

Dumbbell Power Cleans

Step-by-step instructions:

1. Stand with your feet shoulder-width apart, holding a pair of dumbbells in front of your thighs with your palms facing your legs.
2. Quickly shrug your shoulders and pull the dumbbells up to your chest.
3. Dip your legs slightly and pull your elbows high and outside to bring the dumbbells to your front shoulders.
4. Stand up to the starting position, and then lower the dumbbells back to your thighs.

Muscle focus: Quadriceps, hamstrings, glutes, lower back, traps, and forearms.

Safety tips: Keep your back straight, avoid rounding your back, and make sure to control the weight throughout the movement.

Repetitions and sets: 3 sets of 8-12 repetitions, with a weight that allows you to complete all reps with good form.

Variation: You can also perform clean and press, or clean and squat with dumbbells.

Progression: Increase the weight of the dumbbells or the number of repetitions as you progress.

Dumbbell Hang Cleans

Step-by-step instructions:

1. Stand with your feet shoulder-width apart, holding a pair of dumbbells at your sides, with your palms facing your legs.
2. Bend your knees slightly and keep your back straight. Quickly shrug your shoulders and pull the dumbbells up to your chest.
3. Dip your legs slightly and pull your elbows high and outside to bring the dumbbells to your front shoulders.
4. Stand up to the starting position, and then lower the dumbbells back to your sides.

Muscle focus: Quadriceps, hamstrings, glutes, lower back, traps, and forearms.

Safety tips: Keep your back straight, avoid rounding your back, and make sure to control the weight throughout the movement.

Repetitions and sets: 3 sets of 8-12 repetitions, with a weight that allows you to complete all reps with good form.

Variation: You can also perform hang snatch, or hang clean and press with dumbbells.

Progression: Increase the weight of the dumbbells or the number of repetitions as you progress.

Legs and Glutes

Dumbbell Donkey Kicks

1. Begin on all fours with a dumbbell in each hand.
2. Keeping your core engaged and your back straight, lift one leg off the ground, straightening it behind you as you kick it towards the ceiling.
3. Lower the leg back down to starting position, keeping the foot flexed.
4. Repeat with the other leg.

Muscle Focus: Glutes, hamstrings

Safety Tips:

- Keep your back straight and engage your core throughout the exercise.
- Avoid arching your back.

Repetitions: 10-15 repetitions per leg

Sets: 3-4 sets

Variation: Increase weight of dumbbells as you progress.

Progression: Add ankle weights for increased difficulty.

Dumbbell Figure Four Stretch

1. Lie on your back with both legs bent, feet flat on the floor.
2. Hold a dumbbell in your hands, and place your right ankle on top of your left knee.
3. Hold the dumbbell above your chest, keeping your arms straight.
4. Slowly raise your head and shoulders off the ground, keeping the dumbbell in place.
5. Hold for 2-3 seconds before lowering back down to starting position.
6. Repeat with the other leg.

Muscle Focus: Glutes, lower back

Safety Tips: Keep your lower back pressed into the ground, and avoid twisting your torso.

Repetitions: 10-15 repetitions per leg

Sets: 3-4 sets

Variation: Increase weight of dumbbells as you progress.

Progression: Hold the stretch for longer periods of time.

Dumbbell Skater Hops

1. Stand with your feet hip-width apart, holding a dumbbell in each hand.

2. Jump to the right, landing on your right foot with your left leg bent behind you.
3. Jump back to starting position.
4. Repeat on the left side.

Muscle Focus: Glutes, quadriceps, hamstrings

Safety Tips: Keep your knees slightly bent throughout the exercise, and avoid landing with a straight leg.

Repetitions: 10-15 repetitions per leg

Sets: 3-4 sets

Variation: Increase weight of dumbbells as you progress.

Progression: Increase speed of hops.

Dumbbell Bulgarian Split Squats
1. Stand with your feet hip-width apart, holding a dumbbell in each hand.
2. Step back with your right foot, placing it on a bench or elevated surface behind you.
3. Bend your left knee, lowering your body down towards the ground.
4. Push back up to starting position.
5. Repeat with the other leg.

Muscle Focus: Glutes, quadriceps, hamstrings

Safety Tips: Keep your front knee behind your toes, and avoid letting your back knee touch the ground.

Repetitions: 10-15 repetitions per leg

Sets: 3-4 sets

Variation: Increase weight of dumbbells as you progress.

Progression: Increase height of bench or elevated surface.

Dumbbell Glute Bridges

Step-by-Step Instructions:

1. Lie down on your back with your knees bent and feet flat on the floor.
2. Hold a pair of dumbbells with both hands and place them on your hips.
3. Drive your heels into the floor to raise your hips off the ground, keeping the dumbbells on your hips.
4. Hold for a few seconds at the top and then slowly lower back down to the starting position.

Muscle Focus: Glutes and Hamstrings

Safety Tips:

- Make sure to keep your back straight and avoid arching it throughout the exercise.
- Keep the dumbbells close to your body throughout the entire movement.

- Make sure to keep your hips level and avoid tilting to one side.
- Repetitions and Sets: 3 sets of 12-15 reps

Variation: Single-leg Glute Bridges

Progression: Increase weight of the dumbbells and/or add a stability ball to make the exercise more challenging.

Abs and Core

Plank Dumbbell Rows
Step-by-step instructions:

1. Start in a high plank position with dumbbells in each hand, hands placed directly under the shoulders.
2. Keeping your core tight and back straight, row one dumbbell up towards your ribcage, keeping your elbow close to your side.
3. Lower the dumbbell back down to the starting position and repeat with the other arm.
4. Repeat for desired number of repetitions, alternating arms.

Muscle focus: This exercise targets the back, shoulders, and abs.

Safety tips:

- Make sure to keep your back straight and avoid arching your back.
- Keep your core engaged and your neck in line with your spine throughout the exercise.

Repetitions: 8-12 repetitions per arm, for 2-3 sets.

Variation: To make the exercise more challenging, increase the weight of the dumbbells or perform the exercise on an unstable surface such as a stability ball.

Progression: To progress, increase the number of repetitions, sets, or weight of the dumbbells.

Dumbbell Leg Raises
Step-by-step instructions:

1. Lie on your back with a dumbbell between your feet.
2. Keeping your lower back pressed into the floor, lift your legs off the ground and raise them straight up towards the ceiling.
3. Lower your legs back down to the starting position and repeat.
4. Repeat for desired number of repetitions.

Muscle focus: This exercise targets the abs and lower back.

Safety tips:

- Make sure to keep your lower back pressed into the floor and avoid arching your back.
- Keep your neck in line with your spine throughout the exercise.

Repetitions: 8-12 repetitions, for 2-3 sets.

Variation: To make the exercise more challenging, increase the weight of the dumbbell or perform the exercise with a stability ball under your feet.

Progression: To progress, increase the number of repetitions, sets, or weight of the dumbbell.

Dumbbell Side Bends
Step-by-Step Instructions:

1. Start by standing upright with feet shoulder-width apart and holding a dumbbell in your right hand with an overhand grip.
2. Keeping your core tight, bend your body to the right side while keeping your feet firmly planted on the ground.
3. Return to the starting position and repeat the same movement to the left side.

Muscle Focus:

This exercise focuses on the oblique muscles, the muscles on the sides of the torso.

Safety Tips:

- Make sure to keep your core engaged throughout the exercise to avoid straining your lower back.
- Keep your feet firmly planted on the ground to maintain balance.
- Don't use too much weight, start with a lighter weight and gradually increase as you get stronger.

Repetitions and Sets:

Start with 2-3 sets of 10-15 reps on each side, increasing the weight as you progress.

Variation and Progression:

- Add weight to increase the difficulty level.
- Use a Swiss ball for added stability and to engage your core even more.

Dumbbell Reverse Crunches
Step-by-Step Instructions:

1. Start by lying flat on your back with your legs bent at the knees and your arms extended overhead holding a dumbbell.

2. Keep your core tight, lift your knees towards your chest while keeping your feet together.
3. Slowly lower your legs back to the starting position and repeat.

Muscle Focus:

This exercise focuses on the rectus abdominis, the muscles in the front of the abdomen.

Safety Tips:

- Keep your neck relaxed and avoid straining it by looking up.
- Make sure to keep your core engaged throughout the exercise to avoid straining your lower back.

Repetitions and Sets:

Start with 2-3 sets of 10-15 reps, increasing the weight as you progress.

Variation and Progression:

- Hold a medicine ball instead of a dumbbell for added resistance.
- Place your hands behind your head for added difficulty.

Dumbbell Bicycle Crunches
Step-by-step instructions:

1. Lie flat on your back with your knees bent and hands holding a pair of dumbbells.
2. Extend one leg straight out and lift the other knee toward your chest.
3. As you lift your knee, twist your torso to bring the opposite elbow toward the knee.
4. Repeat this motion, alternating legs and elbows with each repetition.

Muscle focus: This exercise primarily targets the rectus abdominis (six-pack muscle) and oblique muscles.

Safety tips:

- Make sure to keep your lower back pressed into the ground throughout the exercise to avoid straining it.
- If you feel any discomfort, stop the exercise immediately.

Repetitions and sets: Start with 3 sets of 12-15 repetitions on each side. Increase the sets and repetitions as you get stronger.

Variation and progression: To make the exercise more challenging, increase the weight of the dumbbells or hold a weight plate.

Dumbbell Ab Rollouts
Step-by-step instructions:

1. Start in a kneeling position with a pair of dumbbells in your hands and arms straight out in front of you.
2. Slowly roll the dumbbells forward, extending your arms and keeping your arms straight, until you feel a stretch in your abs.
3. Hold for a moment and then slowly roll back to the starting position.

Muscle focus: This exercise primarily targets the rectus abdominis (six-pack muscle) and oblique muscles.

Safety tips:

- Make sure to keep your back straight and neck in line with your spine throughout the exercise.
- If you feel any discomfort, stop the exercise immediately.

Repetitions and sets: Start with 3 sets of 8-10 repetitions. Increase the sets and repetitions as you get stronger.

Variation and progression: To make the exercise more challenging, increase the weight of the dumbbells or hold a weight plate.

CHAPTER V: SCULPTING TECHNIQUES 1

High-Intensity Interval Training (HIIT)

High-Intensity Interval Training, or HIIT, is a type of workout that alternates between periods of high-intensity exercise and periods of rest or low-intensity exercise. HIIT has become a popular form of exercise for people looking to improve their fitness and health in a short amount of time. This type of training is perfect for women who are looking to incorporate dumbbell exercises into their routine. Dumbbells provide versatility, versatility and versatility, which makes HIIT training even more effective.

The principles of HIIT training are based on the Idea that short bursts of high-intensity exercise can provide more benefits than longer, moderate-intensity workouts. HIIT workouts typically last between 20 and 30 minutes and are designed to be challenging and intense. The high-intensity intervals push your body to its limits and can help improve cardiovascular health, increase metabolism, and burn more calories than traditional cardio exercises.

One of the key benefits of HIIT training is improved cardiovascular health. HIIT workouts help to increase heart rate and improve cardiovascular function, leading to a healthier heart and better overall health. HIIT exercises also increase the production of endorphins, which can improve mood and reduce stress levels.

In addition to cardiovascular health benefits, HIIT training can also increase metabolism, making it easier to burn fat and lose weight. HIIT workouts cause an "afterburn" effect, which means that the body continues to burn calories even after the workout is finished. This effect can last for hours or even days, making HIIT a great choice for those looking to lose weight and tone their bodies.

HIIT training can also be customized to target specific areas of the body, such as the arms, legs, chest, and core. For example, incorporating dumbbell exercises into your HIIT routine can help to tone and sculpt your muscles, leading to a more defined physique. By using dumbbells during HIIT, you can target different muscle groups and increase overall muscle strength.

Progressive Overload

Progressive Overload is a principle that is widely used in strength training and refers to gradually increasing the weight or resistance used in exercises over time. The idea behind progressive overload is that as muscles adapt to the stress of a particular weight, they become stronger and more able to handle heavier loads. By continually increasing the resistance, you are able to continue challenging your muscles and making progress towards your goals.

Incorporating progressive overload into your dumbbell exercises can be a highly effective way for women to increase their strength and muscle tone. By starting with a weight that is challenging but manageable and gradually increasing the weight over time, you can avoid hitting a plateau and continue making progress. This is important because as your muscles become stronger, they become more efficient at completing the same movements with the same weight, which means you need to increase the weight to continue challenging them.

Progressive overload is a simple principle to implement. For example, if you are performing bicep curls with 5 pounds, you could aim to increase the weight to 6 pounds the next time you do the exercise. This is a gradual increase, but it is important to avoid jumping too quickly to a weight that is too heavy. Increasing the weight too quickly can increase the risk of injury and can also cause your form to suffer, which can negate the benefits of progressive overload.

In addition to increasing the weight, there are other ways to implement progressive overload into your dumbbell exercises. For example, you can increase the number of reps you perform or you can increase the number of sets you do. Increasing the number of reps or sets can be a great way to challenge your muscles without increasing the weight. This can be especially useful for women who are just starting out with strength training and are not yet able to lift heavy weights.

Progressive overload is an important concept for women who are looking to increase their strength and muscle tone with dumbbell exercises. By gradually increasing the weight or resistance used in exercises, you can continue challenging your muscles and making progress towards your goals. It is important to be patient and start with a weight that is manageable, gradually increasing the weight as you become stronger. By using progressive overload, you can ensure that your muscles are continually being challenged and that you are making progress towards your goals.

Supersets and Dropsets

Supersets and Dropsets are two advanced workout techniques that can be utilized in dumbbell exercises for women to increase the intensity and effectiveness of their training. Supersets and dropsets are used to target specific muscle groups and increase strength, endurance, and muscle tone.

Supersets are a type of workout technique where two exercises are performed back to back without rest. This creates a high-intensity workout that requires the use of both strength and endurance. For example, a woman may perform a bicep curl followed by a tricep extension in a superset. By performing these two exercises back to back, the woman can maximize the amount of work done in a shorter period of time. This results in increased calorie burn and improved muscle tone.

Dropsets are a workout technique that involves performing a set of an exercise, then reducing the weight and performing another set. This creates a high-intensity workout that helps increase strength, endurance, and muscle tone. For example, a woman may perform a set of bicep curls with 10-pound dumbbells, then reduce the weight to 8 pounds and perform another set. This creates a high-intensity workout that helps increase strength, endurance, and muscle tone.

The benefits of incorporating supersets and dropsets into a dumbbell workout for women include improved muscle tone and increased strength. Supersets and dropsets are a great way to target specific muscle groups and increase the intensity of a workout. They also help to increase the heart rate and promote cardiovascular health, which results in a higher calorie burn and improved metabolism. Additionally, supersets and dropsets can also help to reduce the amount of time spent in the gym, making them a great option for busy women who want to maximize their workout results.

Plyometrics

Plyometrics, also known as jump training, is a type of exercise that focuses on developing the muscles' ability to produce maximum power in the shortest amount of time. Plyometrics involves explosive movements that are designed to increase the elasticity of the muscles and improve the ability of the body to store and release energy. These exercises are commonly used by athletes to enhance their athletic performance and by fitness enthusiasts to add a new level of challenge to their workouts.

Incorporating plyometrics into dumbbell exercises for women can provide numerous benefits, including improved explosive power, agility, and overall athletic performance. Plyometrics can also help to increase the intensity of a workout, which can lead to greater calorie burn and improved cardiovascular health. Additionally, plyometrics can help to develop the fast-twitch muscle fibers, which are responsible for explosive movements and are often neglected in traditional strength training exercises.

Plyometrics can be incorporated into dumbbell exercises for women in a number of ways. For example, jumping exercises such as box jumps or plyometric push-ups can be performed using dumbbells to add resistance and increase the challenge. Dumbbell plyometric lunges and squats can also be performed to target the legs and glutes. It is important to note that plyometrics should be performed with proper form and with a gradual progression in intensity to avoid injury.

When performing plyometrics, it is important to warm up properly to avoid injury. A proper warm-up should consist of light cardio and dynamic stretching to loosen up the muscles and increase blood flow. After the workout, a cool-down period is also important to allow the body to gradually return to its resting state and reduce the risk of injury.

CHAPTER VI: MINDFUL TRAINING

Mindful Breathing Techniques

Mindful breathing is an essential aspect of fitness and wellness, and it can be especially beneficial when incorporated into a dumbbell workout for women. When we think about exercise, we often focus on the physical aspect of it – the movements, the weights, and the sweat. But the breath is just as important in achieving the desired results.

Mindful breathing is the practice of focusing on the breath and breathing deeply, with full awareness and intention. This can help reduce stress, increase energy levels, and improve mental clarity. When it comes to physical activity, mindful breathing can also help to improve performance and prevent injury.

Here are some mindful breathing techniques that can be incorporated into dumbbell exercises for women:

Diaphragmatic Breathing: This technique involves breathing deeply from the diaphragm, which is the muscle that separates the chest from the abdomen. To perform diaphragmatic breathing, lie flat on your back with your knees bent and place one hand on your chest and the other on your stomach. Inhale deeply through your nose, allowing your diaphragm to expand and push your stomach out. Exhale slowly through your mouth, pulling your stomach in and compressing your diaphragm. Repeat this process several times until you feel relaxed and calm. Benefits of diaphragmatic breathing include reduced stress and anxiety, improved sleep, and better circulation.

Square Breathing: This technique involves breathing in for a count of four, holding your breath for a count of four, exhaling for a count of four, and holding your breath again for a count of four. Repeat this cycle several times until you feel calm and relaxed. Benefits of square breathing include improved focus and concentration, reduced stress and anxiety, and better oxygenation of the body.

Belly Breathing: This technique involves breathing deeply from the belly, which is also known as the diaphragm. To perform belly breathing, lie flat on your back with your knees bent and place one hand on your chest and the other on your stomach. Inhale deeply through your nose, allowing your belly to expand and push out. Exhale slowly through your mouth, pulling your belly in. Repeat this process several times until you feel relaxed and calm. Benefits of belly breathing include reduced stress and anxiety, improved sleep, and better circulation.

Controlled Breathing: This technique involves breathing deeply and slowly, focusing on the sensation of the breath as it moves in and out of your body. To perform controlled breathing, sit or lie down in a comfortable position and close your eyes. Inhale deeply through your nose and exhale slowly through your mouth. Repeat this process several times until you feel calm and relaxed. Benefits of controlled breathing include reduced stress and anxiety, improved focus and concentration, and better oxygenation of the body.

Progressive Relaxation Breathing: This technique involves tensing and relaxing various muscle groups in the body to promote relaxation and stress relief. To perform progressive relaxation breathing, sit or lie down in a comfortable position and close your eyes. Begin by tensing your feet, then your legs, then your abdomen, and so on, until you have tensed all of the major muscle groups in your body. Hold the tension for a few seconds, then exhale and release the tension in each muscle group, starting with your feet and working your way up. Benefits of progressive relaxation breathing include reduced stress and anxiety, improved sleep, and better circulation.

Equal Breathing: This technique involves breathing in and out at the same pace, which helps to calm and focus the mind. To perform equal breathing, sit or lie down in a comfortable position and close your eyes. Inhale deeply through your nose, counting to four in your mind. Exhale slowly through your mouth, counting to four in your mind. Repeat this process several times until you feel calm and relaxed. Benefits of equal breathing include reduced stress and anxiety, improved focus and concentration, and better oxygenation of the body.

Alternate Nostril Breathing: Alternate Nostril Breathing is a simple but powerful breathing technique that helps to balance the body and mind. To perform this technique, sit in a comfortable position and hold your right thumb over your right nostril. Inhale deeply through your left nostril, then hold your breath. Release your right thumb and place your right index finger over your left nostril. Exhale through your right nostril, then inhale deeply through the right nostril and hold your breath. Release your right index finger and place your right thumb over your right nostril. Exhale through your left nostril. This is one round of Alternate Nostril Breathing. Repeat this cycle for several rounds, focusing on the rhythm of your breath.

Benefits: Alternate Nostril Breathing helps to calm the mind, reduce stress and anxiety, and improve focus and concentration. It also helps to balance the nervous system and improve respiratory function.

Lion's Breath: Lion's Breath is a powerful breathing technique that helps to release tension and stress from the body and mind. To perform this technique, sit in a comfortable position and inhale deeply through your nose. As you exhale, open your mouth wide and stick out your tongue, making a loud "ha" sound. Repeat this several times, inhaling deeply through your nose and exhaling with the "ha" sound.

Benefits: Lion's Breath helps to release tension and stress, boost energy and vitality, and improve overall respiratory function. It also helps to improve the immune system and increase mental clarity.

Sitali Breath: Sitali Breath is a calming and cooling breathing technique that helps to soothe the mind and reduce stress. To perform this technique, curl your tongue into a tube shape and stick it out of your mouth. Inhale deeply through your curled tongue, then exhale through your nose. Repeat this cycle several times, focusing on the rhythm of your breath.

Benefits: Sitali Breath helps to cool the body and reduce stress, improve digestion and reduce inflammation, and boost mental clarity and focus.

Four-Seven-Eight Breathing: Four-Seven-Eight Breathing is a simple but powerful breathing technique that helps to calm the mind and reduce stress. To perform this technique, inhale deeply for a count of four, hold your breath for a count of seven, then exhale for a count of eight. Repeat this cycle several times, focusing on the rhythm of your breath.

Benefits: Four-Seven-Eight Breathing helps to reduce stress and anxiety, improve sleep, and boost mental clarity and focus. It also helps to regulate the nervous system and reduce blood pressure.

Ujjayi Breathing: Ujjayi Breathing is a rhythmic and controlled breathing technique that helps to calm the mind and increase focus. To perform this technique, inhale deeply through your nose, then exhale through your nose while making a soft "ahh" sound. Repeat this cycle several times, focusing on the rhythm and sound of your breath.

Benefits: Ujjayi Breathing helps to calm the mind, reduce stress and anxiety, and improve focus and concentration. It also helps to regulate the nervous system and improve respiratory function.

By incorporating mindful breathing into a dumbbell workout, women can improve their physical performance, reduce stress levels, and increase overall well-being. The benefits of mindful breathing are numerous, and it is a simple yet effective way to enhance any workout routine.

Visualization and Affirmations for Improved Performance

Visualization and affirmations are two powerful techniques that can help individuals achieve improved performance and greater success in their endeavors. Visualization involves creating a mental image of a desired outcome or goal and focusing on this image as if it has already been achieved. By doing so, individuals can train their minds to believe that success is attainable and increase their motivation to work towards this goal.

Affirmations are positive statements or declarations that individuals make to themselves to help shape their beliefs and attitudes. These statements can help to increase self-confidence and reduce negative self-talk, which can often sabotage success. By repeating affirmations regularly, individuals can help to rewire their brains and build a more positive and resilient mindset.

When applied to dumbbell exercises for women, visualization and affirmations can be incredibly effective. For example, women can use visualization to see themselves as strong, confident, and capable of achieving their fitness goals. They can use affirmations to reinforce these positive beliefs and declare to themselves that they are capable of success.

The benefits of using visualization and affirmations in conjunction with dumbbell exercises for women include improved motivation and self-confidence, increased focus and concentration, and reduced stress and anxiety. By incorporating these techniques into their workouts, women can achieve greater success and satisfaction in their fitness journeys.

Final Thoughts

As we come to the end of this journey, we hope that you have learned something new and valuable about dumbbell exercises for women. Whether you are a seasoned fitness enthusiast or just starting out, we believe that the information and techniques covered in this book will help you achieve your fitness goals and lead a healthier, more active lifestyle.

We cannot stress enough the importance of proper form and safety when working with dumbbells, and we encourage you to always use caution and listen to your body when performing exercises. Remember, the benefits of dumbbell training go far beyond physical strength and appearance. The mind-body connection and breathing techniques we have discussed will help you feel more relaxed, focused, and confident, both in and out of the gym.

We hope that this book has inspired you to get started on your own journey towards a fit and healthy body. Remember, the only limit to your progress is the one you set for yourself. With persistence and determination, you will see results, and we wish you all the best on your fitness journey.

Continuing Your Dumbbell Journey

As you finish reading this book on dumbbell exercises for women, it's important to remember that your journey to a healthier and more fit lifestyle is not over. The information provided in this book is just a starting point, and there is still so much more to learn and explore when it comes to dumbbell training. In this chapter, we will discuss some tips and strategies to help you continue your dumbbell journey and achieve your fitness goals.

Consistency is Key

One of the most important things to remember when it comes to achieving your fitness goals is consistency. It's easy to get excited about starting a new workout program, but it can be challenging to stick with it in the long term. The key to success is to make your workouts a regular part of your routine and to stick with them even when you don't feel like it. This could mean setting aside a specific time each day for your workout or scheduling your workouts in advance to ensure you stick to them.

Variety is the Spice of Life

It's important to keep your workouts varied and interesting to avoid boredom and plateauing. One of the great things about dumbbell exercises is that there are so many different types of exercises to choose from. You can switch up your routines by using different types of dumbbells, incorporating new exercises, or trying different workout programs. Additionally, you can try combining dumbbell exercises with other types of workouts, such as cardio or yoga, to create a well-rounded fitness program.

Listen to Your Body

When it comes to working out with dumbbells, it's important to listen to your body and know when to push yourself and when to rest. Overworking your muscles can lead to injury and burnout, so it's essential to give your body the time it needs to recover and rebuild. You should also be mindful of any pain or discomfort you may feel during your workouts and adjust your routine accordingly.

Track Your Progress

One of the best ways to stay motivated and see the results of your hard work is to track your progress. You can keep track of your progress by recording your weights, sets, and reps, or by taking before and after photos. This can help you see how far you've come and how much stronger you've become.

Printed in Great Britain
by Amazon

42456918R00066